"Do not be anxious about anything, but in every situation, by prayer and petition, with thanksgiving, present your requests to God."

PHILIPPIANS 4:6-7

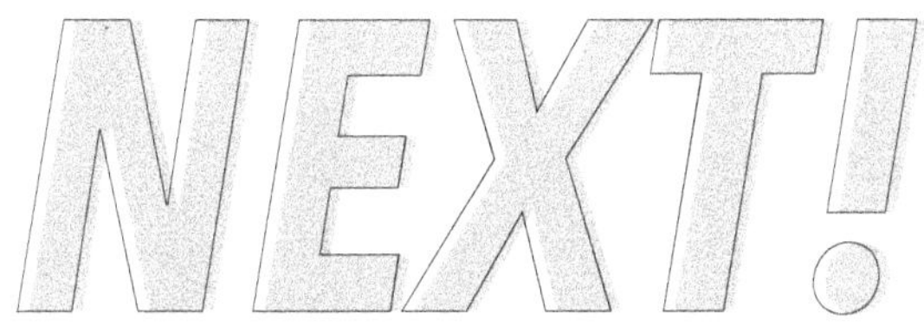

NEXT!

HOW TO KEEP MOVING TOWARD HAPPINESS WITH ONE WORD

STEPHANIE PALMER

Performance Publishing
McKinney, TX

ISBN: 978-1-961781-15-3

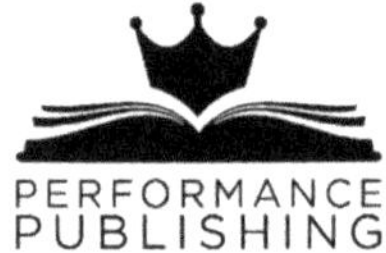

PRAISE FOR NEXT!

Day in and day out, Stephanie shares her secrets to benefit others at great personal sacrifice. She is deeply passionate about inspiring others to achieve what she has through her dedication and perseverance for a better life. She has helped the masses and will continue to do so through the raw words she shares in this book. Stephanie is in the business of changing lives, and I am excited to have a book to get her inspiration regularly. Her example has shown me that change is possible. THANK YOU, Stephanie, for your incredible drive to change the world, one decision at a time.

Kimberly Hawkins
Author of ***Lessons Learned Through No Words At All***
Miramar Beach, Florida

Stephanie nailed it! So often we catch ourselves drifting in life with no direction or purpose, just a series of bad decisions that lead us astray. ***NEXT!*** gives you focus and hope that you can change any situation in which you find yourself by focusing on your ***NEXT*** thought, action, and decision to get you back on track. Simple practices of gratitude in the morning or before bed transform the lens through which you see your life. Stephanie gives practical advice that anyone can use to better themselves at this moment, regardless of their age, past mistakes, or where they are in life. ***NEXT!*** keeps you focused on moving forward towards the life you want. It is a perfect recipe for us all to refocus and recommit, even if we find ourselves distracted or off course.

Dori Capretti
Owner and CEO of Balanced Health and Wellness

Stephanie Palmer's book beautifully encapsulates the essence of **NEXT**, a mindset that propels us forward with unwavering purpose and a commitment to living our best lives. Through her own transformative journey, she inspires us to shed doubt, embrace change, and uncover our true passions. **NEXT** isn't just a word; it's a powerful force for self-discovery and growth, and Stephanie's narrative is a compelling testament to its potential.

Michelle Prince
CEO, Performance Publishing
http://www.PerformancePublishingGroup.com

NEXT is a must-read. It's honest, practical, and inspirational. Palmer shares with her readers a gem she discovered on her journey towards fulfillment. Her technique is universally applicable to any and every aspect of one's life. I highly recommend incorporating Palmer's personal insight on how to find fulfillment in life.

Beth Cameron Scott
Cameron Coca-Cola Family
American Greetings Representative

We have been blessed to be witnesses to the transforming power of what Stephanie describes as her ***NEXT***. Praying your ***NEXTs*** will propel you into positive, life-affirming journeys, too.

Jeff and Julia Igims
Public School Educators for 25+ Years

When people ask me why I am so positive, never appear stressed, and am always in a good mood, my quick is answer that I'm free: free from judgement, animosity, and anxiety. My secret is reading ***inspirational and uplifting*** books like this one. Thank you, **Stephanie**, for sharing a very well-written, to-the-point, educational, inspirational, and empowering, uplifting book. I will add to my weekly mind gym routine.

Gino Chiodo
Co-Owner, Izzazu Salon
Owner, Ruby's Wine House

DEDICATION

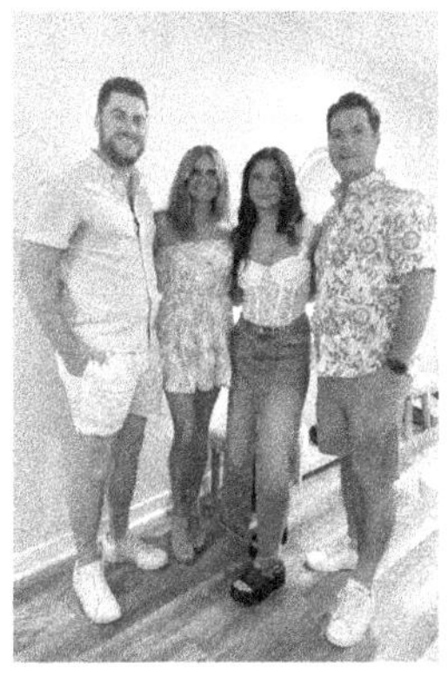

To my husband and the love of my life, Mark, who always knew I had a PASSION inside of me and encouraged me to find it. I love you and am blessed to have you in my life. Also, to my children, Alec and Mia, who are always there to love and support me in all the crazy things I do. And finally, to my parents, Richard and Judy, who have loved me, my siblings, and our entire family unconditionally and have taught me to ALWAYS do the right thing and that EVERYTHING will be okay.

CONTENTS

INTRODUCTION

I love the word *NEXT!* It's a word that keeps us in motion and moving instead of doing nothing. *NEXT* doesn't have room for procrastination or worry. *NEXT* keeps you from focusing on looking back – questioning, doubting, regretting. *NEXT* takes you out of the present and moves you into the future.

The power of NEXT!

I have been on a four-year journey of self-discovery, and I want to share something special, yet simple, with you... a secret way of thinking that has completely changed my life. I know, it sounds gimmicky, but it's not. It is something I learned without even realizing it at the time.

I am challenging my readers to think reflectively for a moment. Is there something about the person you are today that, if you could take a magic wand, you would change right now? I am going to assume that there is, simply because you are human. You can achieve goals, wishes, and dreams that seem out of reach, and I want to inspire you by telling my story about how I finally changed something about myself and how I learned about the power of NEXT.

I did it!

Yes, I am living my best life! It was not the life I planned, but in the end, it is the life that I didn't know I needed. Before I made the change, I was missing a purpose!

As a kid and then a young adult, I did not have any real ambition or drive for anything. No, *my* life plan did not in any way resemble what I found to be my passion later in life. Now that I look back, I can see that all I have ever wanted to do is help other people. My best life centers around my wanting to care for others, starting with my family first; I just did not see it early on. My ultimate purpose took time to unveil itself, and I am so thankful for the results. So, now that I have found my way, I say, "*NEXT!*"

The Starting Point… Searching for More

I went to college because I felt I was "supposed" to go. I was not ready and felt lost in "finding myself," like most people do. My choices were less than productive for my future. It took many years for me to truly find myself and make decisions that would get me back on the right track for me, instead of the track others thought I *should* be on.

Yes, I had my share of problems, and there were more to come. Maybe the problems were not as bad as problems others may have experienced and some were worse than the problems of others; it is all relative, and we need to give ourselves credit for our own personal pains and challenges – instead of comparing. This area is just another way I think people discount themselves – by playing down their struggles.

My problems came about out of my strength and desire to help others. You know how our greatest strength can become our greatest weakness if we get out of balance. Well, that is exactly what happened. It was more than just wanting to help others; I truly had no boundaries regarding what and how I could help. I would just give and give without questioning what it was doing to me or my life.

The challenges I endured led to me *discounting myself and not taking care of myself* rather than designing and living according to my own purpose and the life that I thought I would have. This was the biggest, number one lesson in my life! However, this time gave me a window into the struggle of others that I could not have gained otherwise.

Better Times Ahead

Trying to save the world is exhausting. It took 51 years for me to begin to really take care of ME. Yes, I cared about myself some, but cared about others more. I sacrificed my needs and happiness to help others. Until I found a lifestyle program that transformed the health of both my body and my mind in 2019, I didn't know that I could merge both my need and want to help others – while helping myself first. And this was the beginning of how my purpose and passion began to grow organically.

After making my first "NEXT" decision to try the program, I didn't have the confidence that I would get past one day without quitting, let alone still be going strong coming up on four years. Quitting was MY thing! I had quit most things I'd started. I didn't believe in myself at first, BUT I am here to tell you I surprised everyone. Most importantly, I surprised myself. I became a happy and successful client. It was meant to be!

After I experienced success, I became fully committed. Once I had my "aha" moment that life can be all I dream of and more through the structure of my new lifestyle, I invested in myself and never looked back. After only three-and-a-half months, I lost some unwanted weight, gained positivity and confidence, and found myself again in the journey. I cannot explain what happened to me inside, but I was transformed. I did not only see myself in a new way on the outside, but I had a new view of myself from the inside. I tried things that I never thought I could do and I didn't care about what others thought. I just kept striving for happiness and the key to it all was making my next good decision!

Now, I can show you the way to achieve freedom for yourself, too. It all seems so crazy when I look back at it! When I was ready to move forward, everything changed from the power of one word... *NEXT!*

What will YOU decide at each crossroads of decision making every single day, all day long? I now understand better than ever that I am in control of my happiness and health. It all comes down to the *NEXT* thought, *NEXT* choice, and *NEXT* actions I take.

Focusing on NEXT!

I want to help you find your *NEXT* purpose in this world, just like I did. It's an incredible feeling of freedom when you are always propelling yourself forward instead of living in the past! So, are you with me? Are you committed? Let me show you the way. Say it with me, "*NEXT!*"

CHAPTER 1

How Did I Get *HERE*?

Back when I was a kid, a teenager, and starting college, life was so easy. My parents took such great care of me and my siblings and tried to guide me and teach me all the right things in life. I thought I was on a path that would make them happy until *it* happened! I went from living in my little bubble of bliss protected by my parents to an alternate reality in the big world of the unknown.

When I say *it* happened, it was not just one thing or one event that changed my life; it was a series of choices and decisions that I made and those I did not make along the way. I really thought I knew what life was about and had plans - BIG plans!

My parents and grandparents provided me with the most amazing foundation in life before I went out on my own. They invested in me and showed me what real love looked like - not just in their relationship but in how to treat other human beings. I thought it was just *normal* to live and love the way they did. If I had only known how different the world would be when I went out into it on my own, I would certainly have protected myself much better.

That is how it usually happens though, right? You are going along trying to do what you perceive as your best, when you get knocked down hard. It may be a divorce, an illness, a loss, or even a natural disaster destroying your world. It may even be something that just builds and builds until the tipping point knocks you over.

What happens is not what matters. What matters is that you find your way through it in one piece. What matters is that you learn your intended lessons and persevere. What matters is what's *NEXT!* However it happens, there are answers, and I am here to tell YOU that all you have to do is say, "*NEXT!*"

Struggling and Feeling Defeated

When I think back, I feel bad for that person I was before, but I have no regrets because I have learned so much. Life wouldn't be as good without those lessons. You may think you don't have it in you to even try for a better life. You may think that you have tried everything before, but this may just be your *NEXT!* This one last try may be the last try you need to experience a better life, so don't miss out! Now, say it, "*NEXT!*"

CHAPTER 2

The Wakeup Call

Life is calling, are you answering? Will you answer the call or miss out on the opportunity to see what's NEXT?

You see, sometimes you must take scary and uncomfortable leaps in life. Although they are usually inconvenient, painful, troubling, and outside of your comfort zone, each call can lead you to a better and happier place – eventually.

When I decided to take that NEXT leap to get my life back on track through a transformational health program and then health coaching, I wanted to share it with everyone. I went from working on my health to showing others how to do the same with incredible results! Now, I do it for a living. I found my CALLING, my PURPOSE, my PASSION.

I only wish someone would have taught me these same lessons long ago that I will share with you in these pages. So many years of my life were wasted by being stuck and not being able to make my *NEXT* move. Not only did I find my health through making different NEXT choices repeatedly throughout my day, but I also found meaning in my life and started creating true impact by looking at what is *NEXT* – that NEXT thought, choice, and action!

Whatever it is that is keeping you from living life on fire, the best place to spark the flame is within yourself. Do you tell yourself the lies that you "want" to hear, instead of giving yourself a peptalk of inspiration? Do you say things like these to yourself and others?

- "I am too old to start something new."
- "I am too far gone. Nothing can help me now."
- "I can start that exercise routine next year." (But that day of working out never arrives!)
- "I don't have any talents or passions."
- "I will fail, so why even start?"
- "I know others have done it, but I just cannot follow rules like them."
- "I am too busy."
- "My life is not in a good place right now."
- "I need to focus on my children or spouse right now."
- "I need to wait until things calm down."

Let's face it, life will always have obstacles, so why not decide *now* to make the changes?

A Busy Life

Life is so busy right now that people are being led away from what is important. Isn't it so easy to get off and stay off track? Some people cannot even see the track they are running on currently. Stop and take a breath because your life is about to change!

- Are you someone who lives in frantic chaos all day long, chasing behind all the "to-do's" and spending too much time on the "do not's" in your life?
- Are you working on areas of your life that can create the greatest impact or does that fall off the list day after day?
- Is your life on the right track?

When my life gets a little out of control, that is when I am tempted to lose control – first of my health, and then of other areas. The good news is that one bad decision will not ruin your life, but the culmination of our NEXT bad decision after bad decision over many days, weeks, and months is a different story altogether. The same goes for everything in life. It's making that *NEXT* good decision that can change everything.

So many people feel alone in their troubles, but I am here to tell you that you can succeed and prosper in life. All you must do is take that first step to a better life by believing in yourself and looking at what is *NEXT*! It is all waiting for you!

When I started my journey to a better life through better health, I did not believe it was possible. I had to start working on myself before the belief came to me. Even if it is too much to ask for you to believe in yourself, start your journey anyway. Belief can catch up to you as you see living proof in the results of your efforts.

"A wise man doesn't see his foot on the ground, he watches his NEXT step."

FILIPINO PROVERB

Danger Ahead!

We all have an internal compass guiding us, but sometimes we don't check in with ourselves. We don't think about what NEXT good decision to make. We typically know where the dangers are in life but see something shiny on the other side that we want. We know logically that it is not a good decision but plunge in anyway. Later we feel defeated for making such a poor decision, which makes us victim to yet another poor choice. Then, we sink even lower. Has this happened to you?

It has happened to me, but I've found a way to get back on track by saying, "*NEXT!*" I make small changes that will add up to big results! You can too! How, you ask? Keep reading... *NEXT!*

When we want to build something in life, we must use the same tools to protect ourselves from crumbling. We do this by the choices we make in response to those life-altering events that leave us feeling defeated. We need to move forward - not focused on the future or the past, but really focused on that *NEXT* decision or feeling that will get us through so we can gain strength to move forward. That is what is important, no matter where you are going, focusing on that forward trajectory. Don't live in the past or present! LIVE IN THE "NEXT"!

CHAPTER 3

The Pile On

So, what's NEXT???

Talk to me! How long have you been carrying around extra weight? No, I am not talking about the body weight, but the mental weight you have piled on yourself over the years. Do you even remember what it feels like to be free – free of the weight burdening your body, mind, and soul? How long have you put yourself last or beat yourself up about something over which you have no power? Days, months, years?

The years have a way of collecting baggage, disappointment, rejection, neglect, betrayal, shame, and every other kind of hurt out there. The baggage can pile on us in many forms that typically end in illness, distracting us from fulfilling our potential both physically and mentally. Worse yet, we may just want to hide or escape from life when things are perceived as impossible, unrelenting, and lonely.

In my job as a health coach, I try to create a safe environment for people to share how their life got off track and what led them to this troubled space where they need support. The stories all look a little different, but they all have a thread of similarity to them. We walk through their journey together as they struggle to get their old self back and reach their goals. We look at what is *NEXT* for their lives. I try to teach them how to make their NEXT choices and decisions positive.

This is something I take great pride in today, as it is my goal with each new coaching encounter. I regret that it took me too much time to get to this place where I have the understanding and compassion from my own life experiences to help others. I didn't know this would be my purpose when I started my own journey, but I strengthen in this area every day. As my clients grow, I grow. I have so much gratitude to those who have entrusted their health and lives to me, and I am grateful!

Time to Invest

No, I do not have everything figured out in life. Yet, I have a heightened level of awareness on how to continually advance myself and my life, to do the NEXT best thing so that others around me can do the same. It took me many years to know the key to making others better is starting with making myself better. In order to make ourselves better, investment is required. Until we are willing to invest in ourselves, nothing within or around us can get better.

This means that we must take care of our body, mind, and soul. This will happen through our *NEXT* thoughts, decisions, and actions.

> ... What do I want to eat *NEXT* that will keep me on my path to a healthier life?
> ... What do I want to say *NEXT* when someone is mean, angry, or confrontational with me?
> ... What do I want to do *NEXT* when I run into obstacles that will try and take me away from my goals?

When you live thinking what is *NEXT*, you are always moving forward and, therefore, not looking back. Are you ready to move forward with me?

Let's get started! *NEXT*, please!

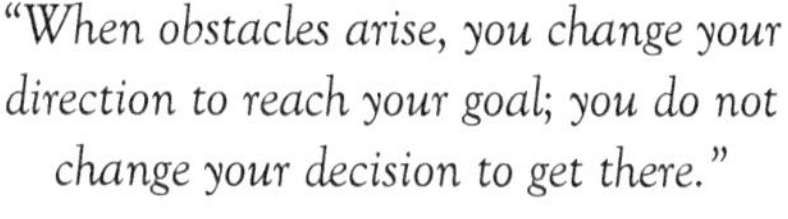

"When obstacles arise, you change your direction to reach your goal; you do not change your decision to get there."

ZIG ZIGLAR

CHAPTER 4

The NEXT Mindset

The NEXT mindset is all about living with the belief that you can have a better life through the choices you make in each moment. Are your NEXT choices making you stronger, healthier, more prosperous? Alternatively, are your NEXT choices leading to pain, disease, obesity, or premature death? It is all up to you!

It may not feel like you have a choice to be where you are in your health, in your relationships, in your job, in your career, spiritually, mentally, etc., but I like to use just one word that will push you ahead… *NEXT!* What is that *NEXT* choice that can change your life? What is that *NEXT* thought? What is that *NEXT* action?

- Will it set you back or propel you forward toward your goals?
- Will it allow you to make progress in your life or drag you down?
- Will it allow you to follow your passion or keep you stagnant?
- Does it make you feel empowered or overwhelmed and defeated?
- Are you finding your true self or burying the real you?
- Are you surrounding yourself with people who are inspiring you to do, be, and gain more out of life? Or are you letting the same people suck the life out of you over and over?

Living with a *NEXT* mindset allows you to pull yourself away from bad choices, decisions, thoughts, and actions, by taking you immediately out of a situation to a positive place with countless possibilities – a place where you can create purpose, passion, and a positive lifestyle.

That NEXT Choice

When I make a poor health decision, I know I can make a better one *NEXT*. Instead of throwing in the towel and going backward, I say, "*NEXT!*" The *NEXT* choice I make will move me closer to my goal, not further from it. Letting go of the poor decision to focus on the *NEXT* decision keeps me motivated and on track overall.

After a few months of making the better NEXT choices in my life, I realized I was in fact digging myself out of the big hole. That hole was burying me and making me unhappy. Once I had developed good habits and a routine with structured support to fall back on, I was able to see everything in my life so clearly. Even on the bad days when I want to give up, I always have *NEXT!* Yes, that NEXT thought, choice, and action!

"Never look down to test the ground before taking your next step; only he who keeps his eye fixed on the far horizon will find the right road."

DAG HAMMARSKJOLD

Let's explore your *NEXT* together.

Starting out the day thinking about what's *NEXT* in life suddenly seems less stressful and more *in the moment*. We are no longer forced to worry about the mistakes of yesterday because we can change our life starting with the choices we are making today. Now, let's get started on what is *NEXT* for you!

Let's Start with the Morning Routine...

There is nothing more important in your day than those first few moments in the morning. You can wake up refreshed and ready to go or tired and wanting to pull the blanket over your head. What will your NEXT decision be? To get up and be happy, accomplish your goals for the day, or go back to sleep and wind up exactly where you are again tomorrow?

I challenge you to start your day strong by taking a few moments to do the following:

- Be grateful and think positive. Thank God for starting you out on a beautiful day (even if it is rainy).
- *NEXT* - this is where you begin those important steps that will further you to a better life or reaching your goals. You could have gotten up and started thinking negatively about how bad everything is, but I'm saying STOP and let your *NEXT* thought be positive.
  - o More importantly, open your eyes with gratitude in your mind and heart. Give thanks!

NEXT

Journal or read a devotional or affirmation that you have made for yourself:

- Clearing your mind can clear out the toxicity within. Find a few minutes to journal your thoughts.
- After you clear your mind and are on the right track, it is time to fuel your body for the day with healthy food and drink.
- Start out by drinking an eight-ounce glass of water. Then choose the healthiest food to start your day.
- If you are feeling really inspired and need a little physical activity, let's get your heart pumping. Take a few minutes to do some exercises. It may be push-ups and sit-ups or just stretching.

NEXT

Gain direction for the day:

- Now that you are fresh and your mind and body are clear, it is time to gain focus. Write down your goals for the day.
- Now focus on those goals. It is important to write down what you will do today to advance in your goals. Each new day, reflect on what you accomplished the day before.

NEXT

Stick to that to-do list and while you are doing it, be kind and encourage others along the way, including yourself!

- Cross each goal off your list as you do it.
- Give someone a compliment or some positive reinforcement – making someone else

feel good has an amazing effect on you as well.

- If you can't accomplish all that is on your list, do what you can and give yourself grace.

You may be thinking, *well, that was easy enough. Is that all I must do?* Well, if you make that one change to incorporate those activities into your life first thing in the morning, then *YES*, life will improve. However, I am here to get you to *the NEXT* level.

If you are like I am and have gone full force ALL day long, frantically running around, it may be difficult to slow down in the evening. So, I take it easy and focus on what is important to me. Before going to bed, the following practices can really change your life for the better:

- Sit down and make a list of everything you will want to accomplish the next day. This will get it off your mind and allow your brain to start to settle down.

- Clean up around you so that you can relax without clutter.
- Read, listen to softer music, call a friend or loved one and make them feel special, or just sit in silence for a few minutes.
- Have gratitude: Close your eyes with a focus on appreciation in your mind and heart. Give thanks!

CHAPTER 5
The Clock Is Ticking

What is *NEXT*?

All of us have a ticking clock, so time is of the essence. We must stay focused on the *now* but live for our dreams of a better *future* by being intentional about what we do *today*.

Nowadays, I am looking ahead and understanding more and more how fleeting our lives can be. With that in mind, I make time for the important priorities in my life, even when I tell myself that there is no time for this or that. The way I define success is by my level of happiness, love, and the quality time I get to spend with my family and my God. They are my foundation, so I invest in them. What do you want to invest in? We must love generously, forgive abundantly, and take great risks.

Your Next

It is your time!

As I close out this book, I want to leave you with one last note to file away for when you need it: When you think 'all or nothing' a lot of the time, you end up with nothing! Don't limit yourself in this way. It is self-sabotage, is defeating, and stops you from going to your *NEXT* level in life. Too many clients of mine don't give themselves the grace and understanding that we all mess up from time to time. It happens! The goal is to go from the mess-up to a leg up by making the NEXT decision – a better one next time – and then pressing *REPEAT!*

The point is to create a new perspective around making your *NEXT* decision a positive one for a better life for yourself. If you can just focus on the *NEXT* time you decide to make a better decision, you will feel empowered, not overwhelmed or defeated. When you make a large or small bad decision in life, there is always that NEXT decision coming at you, allowing you to make a better decision that can change your life repeatedly.

"If nothing changes, nothing changes. If you keep doing what you're doing, you're going to keep getting what you're getting. You want change, make some."

COURTNEY C. STEVENS,
THE LIES ABOUT TRUTH

If you want to know how I do it, I have found that the following principles help me create my best life, full of impact and meaning. I think they will do the same for you.

<u>My Principles to Live By:</u>

- Do not give up!
- You are worth it. Keep it up!
- Have gratitude every day! Start and end your day with gratitude, as well as all the moments you can in-between!
- Reset and start over in life; make your NEXT one better than the last!
- One poor decision does not define you. Let it go and move forward with a focus on making that NEXT decision in life a good one!
- No matter what happens, choose the most positive perspective you can.
- All these NEXT decisions add up over time into a good life!

Prioritize and value yourself or no one else will!

- Find a few things you can be grateful for within you.
- Give yourself a gift for accomplishments of milestones towards your goals.
- Forgive yourself like you would forgive your child, parent, spouse, or best friend.

Find or create structure in your life to help you stay on track with good decisions!

- Set a schedule for eating, drinking water, working, running errands, sleeping, and healthy movement.
- Write down your goals and the steps to get there. Remind yourself of the goals and focus on the one next step to achieve them.
- Surround yourself with people who will inspire you, call you out, and push you out of your comfort zone.

- Giving and feeling unconditional love to and from others is powerful, especially when we find it hard to give it to ourselves.

It Is Time!

If you are looking for more meaning and joy in your days, consider the little pieces of advice in this book. I feel on top of the world most days and want others to experience life just as joyfully as I do. I am giving back to all who gave to me through sharing the building blocks I developed and maintained to get me to a place of greater impact according to my purpose.

I am here to tell you that there is so much more than you can imagine. It is waiting for you! Just get started today! Start by asking yourself, "Okay, what is *NEXT?*"

I am just a normal person who created an abnormally wonderful life by taking a chance on and believing in myself. I have a proven plan that can work for you too, no matter your starting place in life. Let's do it!

What is your *NEXT*??

ABOUT THE AUTHOR

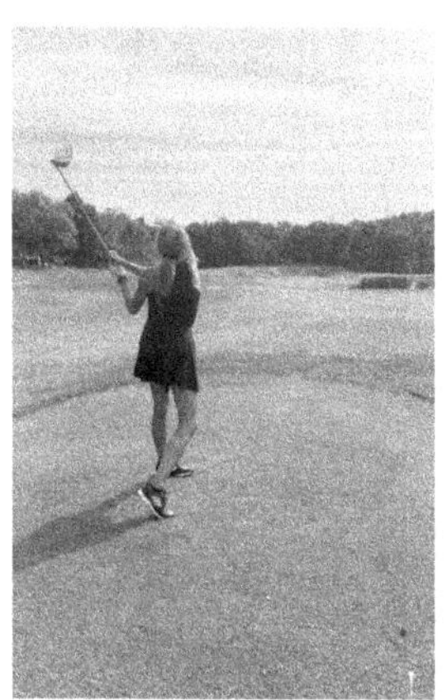
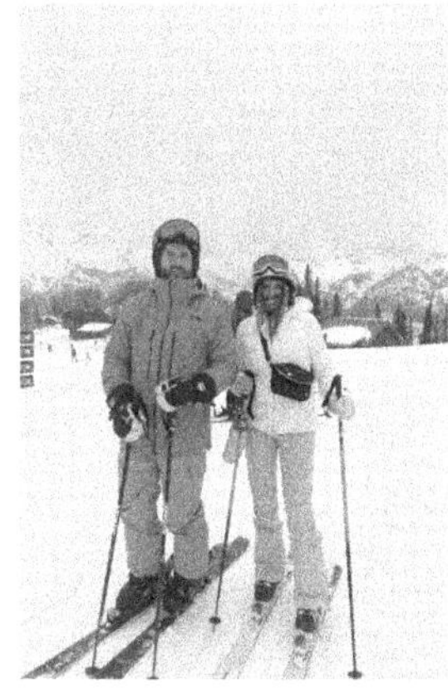

From life shifts to learning new lifts – my 'NEXT' included taking on golf swings and ski slopes.

Stephanie Palmer is a health and wellness entrepreneur who is focused on helping her clients find their "old self" again through personal transformation both physically and mentally. Stephanie has had several "jobs" in her life that range from waitressing to account executive to managing teams across the country. Working with some amazing companies like Coca-Cola, Ecolab, and even Nike, she has always felt that everyone is important, no matter what title they carry or what they do in life and treats everyone with respect.

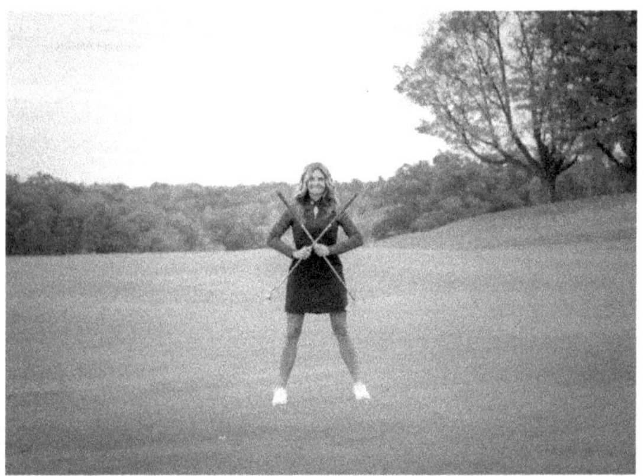

Photo Credit: Erica Sue Photography

Despite her achievements, nothing has brought her as much joy and purpose as when she stumbled, at

51 years old, into a career in which she was able to use her passion to help others, her creativity, and her love to encourage people to gain a new perspective on life by coaching them to become healthy in their mind, body, and soul. For years, starting in college at the University of Pittsburgh and after moving seven times in seven years around the country, she was trying to find the perfect life, the perfect job, and the perfect relationship just like everyone else. She fell into some hard times dealing with a detrimental relationship that was dragging her down to the point where she did not have confidence to pull herself out. With the support of her family and friends, she found her way back to her hometown and made a new start after meeting the love of her life, her husband Mark. Bringing a child into this relationship and finding the person of her dreams were just the start of making her NEXT good decisions to fulfill her life. But, although everything around her was going well, she still lacked confidence and value in herself and felt that she could not find something to

be passionate about. And then, just when she least expected it, it fell into her lap.

What was it? A new lifestyle that changed her life so much that she wanted to help others change theirs.

Stephanie grew up in a very close-knit family in Carnegie, a suburb of Pittsburgh. She was always surrounded by her loving immediate and extended family and has a strong faith and relationship with God. Her parents and grandparents taught her love and respect. There is nothing that makes her happier than serving others and making them feel special and happy.

What she didn't realize was that getting herself healthy and happy would allow her to make a difference in others' lives, which was ultimately her goal and passion.

Stephanie continues to find ways to grow and make both herself and others better, which is evident in her latest endeavor of writing a book and becoming an author. It was a dream and goal that had once seemed unattainable, but through her personal growth over the last four years and coaching others through their individual journeys, it became a reality. She pushes herself out of her comfort zone daily in hopes of having that next person or client find themselves like she found herself. It's never too late to make changes, no matter what age you are or where you come from. She proves that in her own transformation.

Stephanie's hobbies include travel, golf, skiing, and spending time at the beach. Most importantly, she values spending as much time with her husband, Mark, their son Alec and daughter Mia, and the rest of her family as possible.

The biggest joy in her life is to make a difference in someone else's life. Writing this book has been a dream come true.

www.ingramcontent.com/pod-product-compliance
Lightning Source LLC
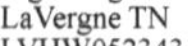
LaVergne TN
LVHW052343100826
845147LV00021B/1169

* 9 7 8 1 9 6 1 7 8 1 1 5 3 *